Healthy Lifestyle for a Healthier You

A Complete Exercise and Diet Plan to Target

Your Body Fat Along With Few Delicious

Recipes

By

Cheryl Green

Book Description

The idea of this book is to present a framework that covers all aspects of healthy eating. The text rekindles the methods and the exercises that can be used to stay healthy and avoid obesity. With fast moving world there has been experienced a great change in food representations. Flavors are given more priority on nourishment. Junk food and fizzy drinks have become our daily food consumption elements. Everyone has accessibility to these foods.

Group of people going for a dine out do not think about what impact they would have after eating certain food, they are ready to spend their incomes on any new variety of food they have heard off. People are running blindly for taste and flavors, this all is very dangerous and is the key aspect of obesity in most of the countries specially

America.

Balanced nutrition and regular exercise are good for your health, even if your weight never changes. Try to set goals that can be accomplished, such as making t small diet changes listed in this book or walking more in your daily life.

With all these things being said we know that one needs proper plan and motivation to start workout. It is not difficult to do however consistency is difficult to maintain.

To keep things easy I have focused on the basic nutrients their source and their amount in one course of meal. This book will surely give you complete guidance and improve your eating habits and fitness issues.

The book is divided into eight sections each of which will give you comprehensive overview of its title. I will gradually start with the introduction and importance of health and fitness progressing towards the key areas and resources that can be used in the process of making our body fit. You will be learning interesting facts and techniques about how to maintain your physical health.

- Introduction gives you the detail about importance of human life and how to stay healthy. It will also get you familiar with terms like calorie count and amount of calories needed by particular age group.

- Chapter one introduces concept of obesity and how it can be avoided. Major vitamins and minerals and their source are also written in detail.

- The next chapter discusses components of fitness along with warm-up exercises of body both at beginners and professional level.

- Chapter three indicates how to get rid of excessive fats from your belly, buttock, and back. The exercises are list down in the chapter.

- Chapter four details the facts about how we are getting excess fats on arms, chin and chest. Result oriented exercises are listed down.

- Chapter five introduces some shakes and smoothies as a best replacement to meals.

- Chapter six introduces some tact's to speed up weight loss either through diet or exercise.

- Finally concluding the book some motivational and healthy tips are given to avoid obesity and lead a happy and fit life.

Introduction

Foundation of human life lies on health. Health is the key element of human life. If you are eating balanced and healthy food only then you are able enough to carry out your routine activities. Healthy food is natural and basic need of human life.

In order to look fresh and beautiful the first thing you should do is to have a keen look on your diet along with your routine. Intake of water and fruits is also an important aspect which should never be ignored.

Great nourishment is one of the keys to great wellbeing. You can enhance your sustenance by making it your routine to eat balanced diet that have a considerable measure of vitamins and minerals in them, for example, vegetables, organic products, grains and low-or

nonfat dairy.

Now I will be discussing some key elements of food, it will give you

the basic knowledge so that you can get the idea about these terms

and their importance in healthy life style:

Calories

The quantity of calories in your daily course of meal is an estimation of the measure of energy that it contains. It is unit of energy. Your body utilizes calories from your meal for activities like strolling, breathing, thinking and other critical capacities. The normal individual needs to consume around 2,000 of calories consistently to keep up their weight, but a man's particular every day calorie count can fluctuate subject to their sexual orientation, age, and physical action level.

Men by and large need a greater number of calories than ladies, and individuals who exercise in routine requires more number of calories than individuals who don't. Even with all these facts calorie count is an important element for kids, elders, men and women. It keeps on realizing you about how much you have ate and how you are going to

burn the rest of extra calories to avoid weight gain or obesity.

The table below is designed to give you an overview of routine calorie

consumption with regard to different age groups and physical level of

people. The values are not fixed, these are estimations based on

results of well reputed health organization in USA.

Category	Age	calories
Active men	14 to 30	2800 to 3000
Inactive men	14 to 30	2000 to 2600
Active women	14 to 30	2200 to 3000
Active men and	Over 30	2200 to 3000

women		
Inactive women	14 to 30	1800 to 2000
children	2 to 8	1000 to 1400
Inactive men and women	Over 30	1800 to 2200

Daily calorie from different sources of food are of vital importance just like the calorie count is important to notice for your every meal. Try to avoid eating unhealthy or "empty calories". It provides you with no nourishment and are source of accumulating extra fats in your body. It comes mainly from solid fats and sugars like such as butter and other dairy products.

A survey result shows that the amount of empty calories comes from the following foods that has become our source of pleasure to eat. These foods are:

Cakes, pastries, buns, doughnuts, sausages, pizza, cream pastas, instant energy drinks, cookies, petties etc.

Chapter 1 – healthy diet to say bye to obesity

Obesity:

Obesity can be referred as state of person's body with an excess of consumed fats and carbohydrates. Obesity is hard to handle or get rid of without proper diet plan and dieting. It also leads to several life taking diseases as discussed below. There is no age restriction for obesity. It can appear to any age group. Fast food, carbonated drinks and unbalanced diets are the main cause leading to obesity. In America 30% of school going children are facing obesity because they tend to like fast food more than fresh fruits and vegetables. Many schools have now put a ban on eating fast food during lunch break, instead they are providing kids with notorious meals.

Body Mass Index:

BMI is a unit to measure body mass. It is common assumption that people with BMI of 30 or more are suffering from obesity. Over fat consumption not only increases your likelihood of having diseases like hypertension, diabetes, sleeplessness, to name a few but it also shatters your self-confidence and makes you feel uncomfortable with response of other people towards you. Majority of people are suffering from obesity and ignoring this fact, they continue with their eating habits.

Measuring obesity through Body Mass Index (BMI) is the common method but it is not the accurate one, we can also measure obesity by checking the waist of person in inches. But again it is not the perfect method. Besides all, these two techniques are commonly used for measuring obesity by doctors. Obesity can easily be judged by appearance but the one who is suffering from it will not believe on

random talks until he or she are told with factual details.

balanced Diet or healthy diet:

A diet with all nourishments and necessary components in meals can be referred as balanced diet. Eating balanced diet in routine is necessary in light of the fact that your tissues +and organs needs appropriate nourishment to work viably. Without proper intake of nutrients, your body is more inclined to contamination, obesity, infections, poor execution and exhaustion.

With rise in population demand for food has terribly increased. Catering these demands many food suppliers and manufactures started to develop grain, fruits and vegetables. Similarly seasonal fruits are grown artificially. These fruits and vegetables are for taste but it does not contain the necessary minerals and nutrients needed by our body.

The problems of health and several diseases like diabetes and heart strokes in USA is mainly caused by artificial foods. This also leads to abnormalities in physical as well as metal state of man. The health authorities in America reported that almost 40% of the reasons for death in the United States are straightforwardly affected by eating unhealthy food. According to a survey 20% to 30% of a population are facing these diseases and there has been some cases with toddlers, kids and newborns. These common diseases are:

- Cancer

- diabetes

- heart disease

- strokes

Nutrients and their importance

As discussed before the importance of balanced diet in our lives. Main nutrients and food components you need to take on daily basis to avoid obesity or any related health issue. Following are some food groups that plays vital role in balanced diet:

1. Vegetables

Vegetables are considered as a basic source of necessary minerals and vitamins. Green leafs and Dark colored vegetables usually comprise most of the important nutrients. You should add variety of vegetables in routine meals. Try to use vegetables that are fresh and seasonal. You can also eat vegetables without boiling or cooking it.

Vegetables are source of water intake along with numerous supplements, including potassium, folic acid, vitamins and fibers. Vegetables like tomatoes, broccoli, garlic, and spinach give extra advantages, making your meal a super food!

- Potassium may keep up sound circulatory strain. Dietary fiber from vegetables lessens blood cholesterol levels and may bring down danger of coronary illness.

- Another important vitamin is Folate (folic corrosive). It helps your body in structuring of solid red platelets. It increases your blood flow and strengthens your heart. Ladies carrying a baby in their wombs should have this vitamin as fetus needs folic acid for its neural development and spine growth.

- Vegetables containing folic acid are:

- ➢ collard greens

- ➢ spinach

- ➢ broccoli

- ➢ kale

- ➢ Swiss chard

- ➢ green beans

2. Fruits

Fruits bring ultimate freshness in your skin and improve overall system of your body. Fruits are natural source of nourishments. You should always try to use fresh and seasonal fruits. There are a lot of canned fruits available in markets and a lot of suppliers have started to grow these fruits artificially, try to avoid these. It will only give you taste for few minutes and will not be beneficial at all for your body.

You can make different juices, shakes, salads and even snacks. Make it essential course of your meal in daily routine.

3. Grains

As per the USDA, Americans eat refined white flour more than other grain. But the fact is, refined white flour is poor in nutritious level. It is due to the fact that during process of refining grains from the fields, the frame of the grain is evacuated leaving behind refined grain which is of no use to health. Its nourishment lies in external shell that is usually removed. We can separately add fiber in it after words to increase worth of refined grain. Separate fiber is easily available in markets. This is the reason that most of people have switched from white rice and white breads to brown rice and brown bread. It is healthy to eat these instead of fine grain products. It also helps in digestion of food.

4. Dairy products

Dairy products are best source of providing vitamin D, calcium, and other important nutrients. But we cannot ignore the fact that they have lots of calories and saturated fats that can cause obesity or blockage in arteries. When a person consumes dairy products that are high with fat ratio on daily basis, he is likely to get effected by heart diseases. Recent increase in heart attacks are result of consuming more fats either directly from dairy products or fast food like buns, donuts and pizza which contain 75 % of fats. So to avoid this situation you should take small portions of reduced-fat, full-fat cheeses, and or yoghurt and fat-free milk.

Milks that are obtained from plants like almond milk, flaxseed milk and soy are mostly the rich source of calcium, magnesium and other nutritional vitamins, you can use these milks instead of consuming more fats from dairy products. They offer an excellent alternative to animal's milk.

5. Proteins

Proteins are an essential nutrient in development of human organs. Beans and animal meat are its basic sources. If you have a muscle injury or any physical injury, all you need to do is to add or increase portions of protein in your routine meal. It is vital element for proper brain and muscle development. Meat containing low-fats like fish, chicken, beef and prawns are the best for consumption of proteins.

You can also remove animal fat while cooking it. Try to remove visible fats and the skin; it is an easy way to deduct the quantity of cholesterol and fats in your meal. Try to use fresh meat. There are many chemicals and medicines that are used to enhance growth and to increase or swell meat of animals for commercial purposes. This does not only give birth to contagious diseases like bird flu but are also risky for mental health. So, the diet and health of the animals consumed by common public is important. If animal has consumed chemicals for speedy weight gain then people consuming it will suffer from harmful diseases. The best options for commercial used animals are to grass feed them.

There are also some other sources to consume protein, these may contain remedy for many diseases and many other benefits to health.

Proteins, fiber and other nutrients including beans and nuts like:

- walnuts

- Lentils

- sunflower seeds

- peas

- almonds

- soya beans

- tempeh

- tofu

These beans are all excellent alternative to meat; fish, beef etc. try to consume variety of food so that you can consume best out of it.

6. Oils

Oils are vital part of our everyday meal. Every food whether its gravy, dry nuts, and fried chicken contains oil. So we cannot avoid using it. However we can lessen up its quantity. Try to use low-sugar and low-fat forms of products which contain oils in food such as mayonnaise and salad dressing. There are also plenty of oil types that are good to consume and are termed as good oils like olive oil, can be opted as a best replacement for full of fat vegetable oil in our food. Try to avoid fried foods items because they are rich in empty calories (not beneficial to health).There is an availability of an operational calculator by USDA. It helps in calculating the amount of how abundant of you should consume particular nutrient and vitamins from each food group on routine basis.

Apart from accumulating certain nutrients through food in your diet, you have to work on reducing your ingesting of certain fats and foods to sustain a healthy weight and a balanced diet. These include:

- solid fats

- saturated fats

- salt

- alcohol

- sugars

- refined grains

- trans fats

Moreover you can follow a complete diet plan or concern your doctor or physician for proper guidance. If you have queries regarding your diet or feel that you are overweight and you need to drop few Kilo grams, follow complete instruction and diet plan and you must improve your eating habits. Set up an appointment with nutritionist so he can guide you properly. They can recommend nutritive changes that will benefit you to get the diet you require while improving your health.

Liquids:

So far I have discussed what to eat and all minerals and vitamin but you should also know what drinks you should take and what to avoid.

Tea: It is healthy; it can be used as a cleanser to a body because of its richness in antioxidants with a plus point of having less caffeine in comparison to coffee.

Coffee: Coffee is healthy and very rich in antioxidants, but people who are sensitive to caffeine should avoid it. Avoid coffee late in the day because it can ruin your sleep.

Water: A human body needs plenty of water to stay hydrated. You must drink water during the day and particularly during the workouts.

Fizzy or carbonated drinks without artificial flavors and sweeteners are fine but in small quantity.

Try to avoid fizzy drinks with sugar and artificial fruit juice, sweeteners and beer.

Chapter 2 – Warm up Exercises

Before I discuss the warm-up exercises that should be strictly followed along with balanced diet, I will discuss primary components of health and fitness.

Components of Fitness

The four essential parts that are critical to enhanced your physical wellbeing are as per the following:

1. **Muscular limit** alludes to the range of strong ability. This incorporates strong perseverance of the capacity to apply power over a drawn out stretch of time. Solid quality (i.e., the capacity to create power, or the most extreme measure of power that a muscle can apply

in a solitary compression); and strong force (i.e., the capacity to produce quality response in acritical time). A portion of the long haul adjustments of enhancing strong limit are expanded quality, enhanced solid continuance, expanded metabolic rate, enhanced joint quality, and general stance.

2. Cardiorespiratory limit is the capacity of the body to take in oxygen (breath), convey it to all the cells (flow), and utilize it at the cell level to make energy for physical work (action). Similarly in fitness we allude to cardiorespiratory limit as high-impact limit. This limit incorporates oxygen consuming perseverance (to what extent), high-impact quality and high-impact power. A portion of the long adjustments of cardiorespiratory preparation are: diminished heart rate, diminished danger of cardiovascular sickness, enhanced perseverance and expanded stroke volume.

3. Body arrangement is the extent of fat mass in muscle, bone, blood, organs, and liquids to fat mass in fat tissue stored under the skin and around organs. It is the movement or integrity of all joints working in collaboration with each other.

4. Flexibility is the scope of development or measure of movement that a human joint is equipped for performing. Every joint has an alternate measure of adaptability. A portion of the long adjustments of enhanced adaptability are less harmful. It enhanced scope of

movement, more substantial developments and enhanced stance.

Some other aspects of fitness:

These are performance based or physical components of fitness.

These components are involved in all routine activities of a person

and are essential for routine functioning of body. Athletes or people

who tend to do more physical exertion than normal people experience

physical stability at different levels of routine task depending on how

there body is dealing with these secondary health components. You

should have a basic knowledge regarding these components so that

you can set your diet and do exercise on daily basis to maintain

fitness.

- **Coordination**: it is the capacity of a person to use his all body parts in a composed manner which aid in producing fluid and smooth movement.

- **Speed:** it is the capability of a person to act swiftly. You mental speed or speed in which you respond to particular action or emotion depends on it. Speed can also be referred as velocity with time.

- **Balance:** it is the ability of a person to maintain his posture or specific position of a body in either a dynamic or stationary (static) position.by maintaining your balance you have the capacity to hold your own weight with ease.

- **Reaction time**: it is the response time that a person's mental and physical body takes to act against any stimulus.

- **Agility**: it is capacity of an individual through which it changes its direction of motion in a quick manner.

- **Mental capability:** it is the capacity to stay focused and allow you to concentrate during any physical movement to improvise working out properties and the ability to enjoy and relax the mental state of activity.

- **Power** is gained by both speed and strength. It is the energy utilized by a person to do its routine task efficiently. It is an overwhelming strength that one's feel within himself.

The warm-up exercises

We all want a perfect body shape and physique, but remember this all needs a little attention with routine workout so get ready to stretch your body by following these amazing warm-up exercises. Every day work like picking things, dropping trey balls, walking around the house and cleaning house all day are for sure physical work but proper workout is necessary in order to get your body in shape. Make sure that you do any of these nine effective and fresh warm-up exercises.

- **Jumping**

It is a healthy exercise and can get you warmed up in couple of minutes. Mostly fitness experts' advice to do two consecutive sets of jumping in five minutes. It can be with help of rope or random jumping, but remember to leave your arms free, don't stiff them. Do it in a routine and try to do more sets and increase your exercise time to maximize your capacity.

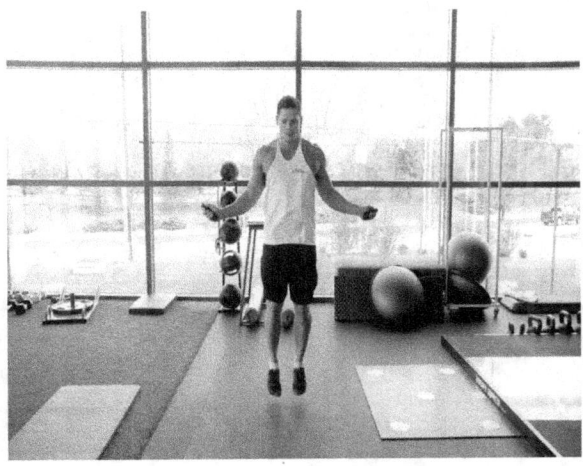

Dynamic movement:

These incorporate activities, for example, the forward rush, sidelong squat, hand walk, or arm circles. After these movement exercises, do directly 3 sets of 15-yard straight skips and after that up with 3 sets of 15-yard Carioca to complete it off. Your body is currently prepared for workout execution!

Functional balance:

Have a one warm-up set of a parity practice that mirrors the genuine preparing practices you'll be doing. This will initiate your body system for exercise. There are some cases that incorporate single-leg deadlifts with a dumbbell in the hand reversing the other leg, or twist around columns while remaining on the level side of your trainer.

Continuously attempt a warm-up set that uses the muscles you have plan to work stabilizing

Legs warm up

This warm up will work your legs, center, and heart all together. Contingent upon your motivation to hardware and objectives, do a 5-to-10 minute warm-up, took after with light extending of the body parts on that day's preparation log. Consider froth rolling the particular zones to expand your execution potential.

Keep in mind, warm-ups are not planned to be a piece of the workouts. Break a brief sweat however don't work so hard that you develop lactic corrosive; spare your vitality and energy for the real workout. Make yourself comfortable through work out, don't get over burden or exhausted by it.

This advances blood stream and prepares your heart for more work. Envision your body as a dragster which is prepared to do a quarter-mile drag at full power, however to satisfy your potential, you have to warm up those slicks and make them pleasant and sticky!

Swinging

Utilizing your warm up session in swinging is an incredible approach to release up your muscles and joints so they are prepared for taking care of substantial resistance.

Your muscles and joints resemble elastic groups - they'll snap when cool, however in the event that warmed up, they'll be versatile, responsive and adaptable.

Have a look on these activities to get ready for an awesome workout.

- Arm Circles: 1 set of 10 reps, advances, 1 set of 10 reps, in reverse

- Straight Leg March: 2 sets of 15 yards

- Cross-Body Leg Swings: 1 set of 10 reps, every leg)

- Arm Swings: 1 set of 10 reps

- Standing Gate- While Walking: 2 sets of 15 yards

- Front to Back Leg Swings: 1 set of 10 reps, every leg

Chapter 3 – Exercises to Target Belly, Buttock, and Back Fat

Belly, Buttock and back are all prominent features of our body. Females and males both are conscious about these body parts, because if you have extra fats on these body parts it doesn't looks good and also turned down your personality.

Exercises to cut down fat from Your Butt, Belly, and Thighs

Tired of the irritating zipper move, you play out every time you wear your most loved pair of pants? All things considered, inspiration and motivation can prepare you to hurdle up effortlessly: these exercises mentioned below have the ideal impact to firm your butt, smooth your midsection, condition your thighs, and impact fat all around.

To prompt genuine body transforms, you should shake up your ordinary routine, Stair climbing right away helps your heart rate and gives an additional strong test. Do the accompanying quality and stair workouts three times each week on nonconsecutive days. Include one bumpy climb or more and keep running on weekends, to impact significantly more calories should be cut down and you'll be slipping into those thin pants in a month or so!

Running

Target: Calves, Hips, Thighs, Core

1. Stand confronting stairs with elbows bowed at sides.

2. Take a mammoth stride up to second step with right foot, then bounce up, bringing left knee toward mid-section.

3. Land on stair with right foot.

4. Immediately venture down to the floor with left foot while bowing right leg behind you.

5. Hold for 5 tallies, keeping your abs tight to help you adjust.

6. Do 16 to 20 hazardous bounces on right foot, utilizing your arms to pick up force; switch sides and rehash.

Fledgling Option: Step up without bouncing; hold the end period of the activity for 2 seconds, touching back foot to floor to help with parity.

Reverse Lunge

Target: Legs, Hips, gluteus

1. Stand confronting staircase with right foot planted on the first or second step, holding 3-to 5-pound weights at hips.

2. Leaning forward marginally, thrust back with left leg, bowing right knee 90 degrees and keeping knee adjusted over lower leg.

3. Remain in low position and convey surrendered foot over to meet right on step.

4. Squat down, bringing down hips another 2 inches. Hold for 2 sec.

5. Do 16 to 20 repetitions, rotating sides.

Amateur Option: Lose the weights and curve knees just 45 degrees.

Do 12 reps on every leg.

Standing Flight

Target: Thighs, Claves, Shoulders, Hips, Core, Chest.

1. Stand sideways to stairs, setting right foot on the first or second

    step.

2. Keep feet wide separated and turn toes out 45 degrees.

3. Hold a 3-to 5-pound dumbbell in every hand, palms forward,

    arms stretched out at mid-section tallness and elbows

    marginally twisted (not appeared).

4. Bring weights together before mid-section while bringing down

    hips into a plié.

5. Hold for 2 seconds.

6. Return to beginning position and rehash for 16 to 20 reps; switch sides.

Starter Option: Lower mostly down into a semi plié; keep hands on your hips (no weights).

Leg-Step Extension

Target: Hips, Hamstrings, Core, Chest, Arms

- Get on all fours with hands stacked under shoulders and toes squeezed into step.

- Tuck right knee in toward mid-section.

- Extend right leg behind you and crush gluteus; hold for 2 numbers (not appeared).

- Do 10 reps; switch sides.

Starter Option: Do this activity on the floor rather than the stairs, and perform just 6 reps for each leg.

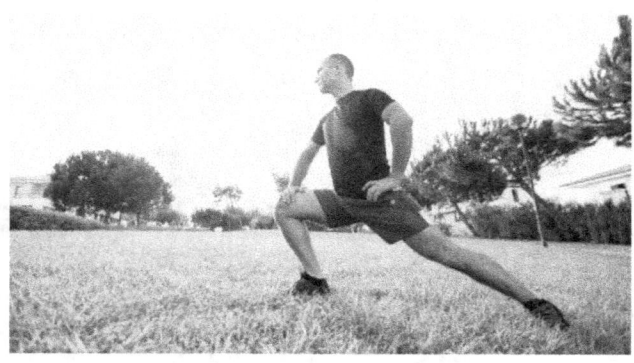

One -Leg Rotation

Target: Hips, Legs, Gluteus, Thighs

- Stand confronting far from the stairs with left toes on the initial step, middle straight, holding a 3-to 5-pound dumbbell in every hand.

- Bend right knee 90 degrees, keeping knee adjusted to lower leg.

- Turn middle to one side and bring weights over outside of right thigh.

- Hold for 2 checks; come back to begin.

- Do 16 to 20 repetitions; switch sides while exercising.

Chapter 4 – Good Bye to heavy arms, Double chin and Chest

I know a number of ladies grumble about their muscle to fat quotients, and particularly about the fat from specific parts of their body, as: under button fat (twofold jaw), midsection fat or armpit fat.

Ladies are usually more conscious about their appearance as compared to men so they also have greater motivational level. I am going to focus on the most proficient method to dispose of armpit fat.

So with a specific end goal to dispose of armpit fat or fat from any parts of the body we need to lessen our muscle to fat ratio ratios generally speaking through practicing furthermore eating an all-around adjusted eating routine. So a full body workout comprises in both cardio and quality preparing. This can decrease muscle to fat

ratio ratios furthermore to dispose of armpit fat.

Compelling Workout To Get Rid Of Armpit Fat

This workout will mean to condition the 'armpit fat' range through

mid-section practices which additionally incorporate your shoulders

and arm muscles. So all you'll need is a couple of moderate weight

dumbbells (4-6 kg each). You can do these activities on a mat, on a

seat or on a Swiss ball which will make it additionally difficult.

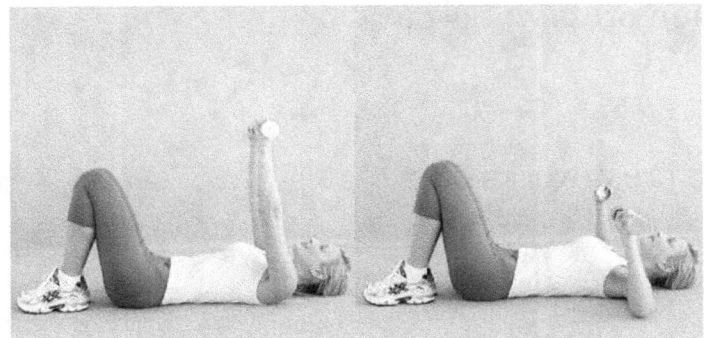

Lie on your back and snatch your dumbbells and lift them up to the roof. Ensure they are in accordance with your mid-section. Keep your knees up and your feet level on the floor. Bring the dumbbells towards your mid-section, gradual. When you touch the floor with your elbows return gradually to the beginning position. This is one rep.

In the course that you need to dispose of armpit fat, you have to perform:

- 10 gradually mid-section press works out;

- 10 rapidly mid-section press works out;

- 5 gradually;

- pulse 10 times (part of the way through);

- Staggered Push Up (16 reps)

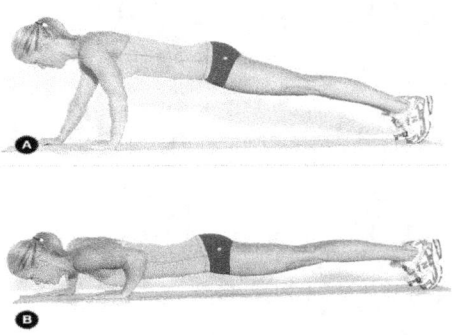

Pushups is one of the best upper body workout and it really tones the entire 'armpit fat' area. Instead of the normal push up, for staggered push up you need to place one arm at the chest level and one arm about 3 inches forward. This will challenge your arm even more. Do 8 reps on each side.

Dumbbell Flies

You have to do dumbbell flies to get rid of armpit fat! It's a must do.

These exercises really work on the exact area you want and definitely will tone it up.

Begin this one from the exact posture just like in the first exercise mentioned above. Your palms should be facing inwards, now open it gently to the point that your upper arm drops on the floor and then cuddle it upwards. Try to mechanize your moves in a slow manner so that ever muscles of your targeted body parts may incorporate in exercise.

Armpit fat make you look bigger and fattier than your age so here are some other useful exercise tips to get rid of this excessive fats:

- 10 slow motion fly exercises.

- 5 slow motion flies.

- 10 quickly fly exercises.

During the exercise try to take rest for one minute or two minutes depending on your strength. Do the exercises in sets and take rest between each set. Repeat the same workout to avoid armpit fat. Do this work out 2 or 3 times in routine along with other work outs. Try to improvise your strength and maintain your stamina. With motivation and consistency, you are going to get your armpit in shape.

Exercise to reduce or enhance chest for women:

The workouts that are associated to chest are the generic ones for both genders. Pushups is considered to be the most effective exercise to work out the complete upper part of your body. It reduces excess fats from your shoulders and triceps. You can make variations in the

exercise depending upon your mood and ease. If you are doing it for

the very first, then begin this work out like simple small pushups with

set of five and gradually increase you capacity to set of ten and so on.

Chapter 5 –Meal Replacement Smoothies

Planning your diet plan toward losing one to two pounds a week gives a protected and solid rate of weight reduction. A dinner substitution smoothie can give breakfast to raise your digestion system when you begin your day. In the start the initial two weeks of calorie diminishment, you may lose more weight, particularly in the event that you perform oxygen consuming practice, for example, power strolling or running most days of the week. Exercise blazes more calories and helps your body put away fats. Oxygen consuming movement likewise helps your vitality, enhances your cardiovascular health, diminishes stretch and supports your state of mind. The advantages of this activity enhancement are that it improves your

mental health and strengthen observance of good diet propensities.

Cutting calories works, weight reduction originates from changing

your calorie count, adjust with the goal that you will burn number of

calories in physical action than you expend. A feast substitution

smoothie, for example, a protein beverage, may help you to devour

less calories to get in shape. Eating an ideal diet in routine and

practicing gives the best procedure to enduring, fruitful weight

reduction. But before trying any of these you should take guidance

from your physician or nutritionist.

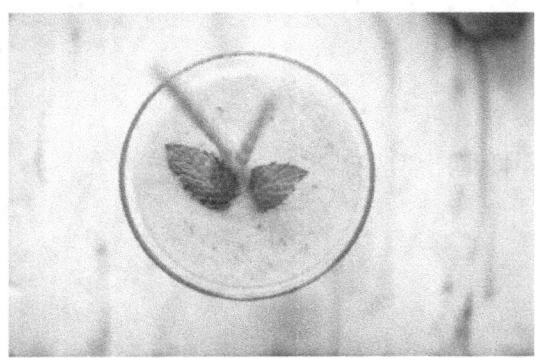

White smoothie:

Here I am going to share a very interesting recipe with you. You will surely observe a difference in yourself if you try it on regular basis with a little bit of work-out.

Ingredients:

2 cups almond milk, preferably unsweetened

2 cups fresh kale

2 cups berries

1 banana

2 tablespoons almond butter and ¼ cup rolled oats

Recipe:

1. Blend almond milk and kale in a blender or shaker until smooth.

2. Add left over ingredients, and blend it well until it is smooth.

3. Add ice cubes to make it feel better.

There are also several shakes and smoothies available in markets that are ready to serve. Some of these are discussed below:

Organic shakes:

In case you are searching for natural flavored shake you can get for your work out, always opt for organic shakes. These shakes come in variety of flavors. Most commonly used flavors are vanilla, chocolate fudge, strawberry and frosted ice cream mocha. One pack of it contains 16 gm of protein made from casein powder. This 11-ounce of shake is composed of 255 calories, 2 grams of fiber and 7 grams fat. You can also add nuts and dry fruits to make it a complete meal replacement smoothie.

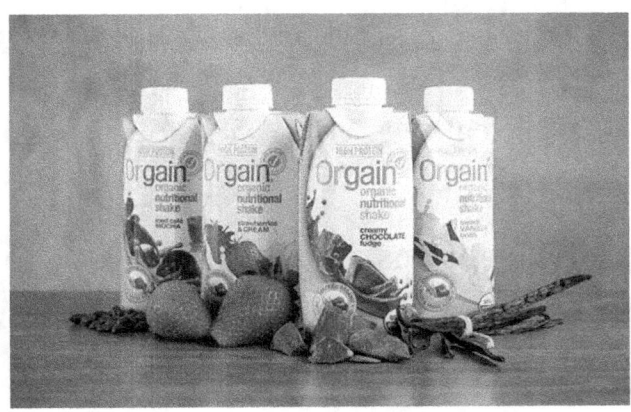

Protein shakes:

Isopure shake are protein rich shakes. Its texture is smooth and good to taste. The best flavor available in markets is alpine punch. It carries 25 gm of crabs and 40 grams of proteins making it a 260 calorie drink. It does not contain any fats or fiber so drink it with chill. You can also add nuts or avocado to add some fats and fiber in it depending upon your need.

EAS Shake

This shake is designed or made specifically as after work out drink. This beverage   can be used as two options. It can be used as a replacement to your meal drink along with it, we can drink it after exercise session. It contains almost 42 gm of proteins obtained from pea powder and whey. If you buy a carton of it remember this that you are buying 300 calories which has ability to satisfy your fats and protein need. You can also use it as dressing or toppings in fruit salads or desserts. Its carton will cost you a maximum of $3 and is available in super markets and stores.

Chapter 6- Healthy Recipes to increase Weight Loss Speed

1. Broccoli & Feta Omelet with Toast

This easy breakfast recipe, which takes just 15 minutes start to finish, packs a one-two punch that will leave you feeling satisfied yet energized.

Ingredients:

Cooking spray

1 cup chopped broccoli

2 large eggs, beaten

2 tablespoons feta cheese, crumbled

1/4 teaspoon dried dill

2 slices rye bread, toasted

Preparation:

1. Heat a nonstick skillet over medium heat. Coat pan with cooking spray. Add broccoli, and cook 3 minutes.

2. Combine egg, feta, and dill in a small bowl. Add egg mixture to pan. Cook 3 to 4 minutes; flip omelet and cook 2 minutes or until cooked through. Serve with toast.

Nutritional Information:

Calories per serving   390

Fat per serving: 19g

Saturated fat per   6g

serving:

Monounsaturated   5g

fat per serving:

Polyunsaturated fat per serving:	2g
Protein per serving:	23g
Carbohydrate per serving:	35g
Fiber per serving:	6g
Cholesterol per serving:	440mg
Sodium per serving:	550mg

2. Banana & Almond Butter Toast

This simple yet tasty morning pick-me-up features no fewer than three of the best foods to eat for breakfast. The bananas and whole-grain rye bread are high in resistant starch, to help boost metabolism, while the almond butter adds hunger-curbing protein and healthy monounsaturated fats.

One slice contains just 280 calories, but it's guaranteed to keep you full until lunchtime.

Ingredients:

- 1 tablespoon almond butter

- 1 slice rye bread, toasted

- 1 banana, sliced

Preparation:

1. Spread almond butter on toast.

2. Top with banana slices

Nutritional Information:

Calories per   280

serving:

Fat per serving:	**11g**
Saturated fat per serving:	**1g**
Monounsaturated fat per serving:	**7g**
Polyunsaturated fat per serving:	**2.5g**
Protein per serving:	**6g**
Carbohydrate per serving:	**44g**

Fiber per serving:	5g
Cholesterol per serving:	0.0mg
Sodium per serving:	260mg

3. *Honey Grapefruit with Banana*

Trying to trim down or stay slim? You can't go wrong with this tangy tropical fruit salad, perfect for breakfast or as a colorful side dish at brunch. Grapefruit is one of the best foods for weight loss, studies show—perhaps because of the effect it has on insulin, a fat-storage hormone.

What's more, grapefruit is deceptively filling. It has one of the highest

water concentrations of any fruit (about 90% of its weight is water),

and all that juice fills you up fast and prevents overeating.

Ingredients:

- 1 (24-ounce) jar refrigerated red grapefruit sections (about 2 cups)

- 1 cup sliced banana (about 1)

- 1 tablespoon fresh chopped mint

- 1 tablespoon honey

Preparation:

Drain grapefruit sections, reserving 1/4 cup juice.

Combine grapefruit sections, juice, and remaining ingredients in a medium bowl. Toss gently to coat. Serve immediately, or cover and chill.

Nutritional Information:

Calories per serving:	122
Caloriesfromfat per serving:	3%
Fat per serving:	0.4g
Saturated fat per	0.1g

serving:

Monounsaturated   **0.0g**

fat per serving:

Polyunsaturated   **0.0g**

fat per serving:

Protein per   **1.5g**

serving:

Carbohydrate per   **31.3g**

serving:

Fiber per serving: **3.4g**

Cholesterol per   **0.0mg**

serving:

Iron per serving: 0.6mg

Sodium per   2mg

serving:

Calcium per   26mg

serving:

4. Breakfast Barley with Banana & Sunflower Seeds

Looking for a healthy start to your day? Tired of oatmeal? Switch

things up with this crunchy breakfast bowl. The combination of barley

and banana provides nearly 8 grams of resistant starch, plus

metabolism-boosting fiber, making this an ultra-satisfying morning meal.

And trust us, it's not nearly as boring as it looks: A spoonful of honey and a sprinkling of sunflower seeds give this hearty dish a delicious sweet-and-salty finish.

Ingredients:

- 2/3 cup water

- 1/3 cup uncooked quick-cooking pearl barley

- 1 banana, sliced

- 1 tablespoon unsalted salted sunflower seeds

- 1 teaspoon honey

Nutritional Information:

Calories per serving:	410
Fat per serving:	6g
Saturated fat per serving:	.5g
Monounsaturated fat per serving:	2g
Polyunsaturated fat per serving:	2.5g
Protein per	10g

serving:

Carbohydrate per   86g

serving:

Fiber per serving: 14g

Cholesterol per   0mg

serving:

Sodium per   15mg

serving:

Resistant starch   7.6g

per serving:

5. Curried Egg Salad Sandwich

Eggs are an ideal food for dieters. They're tasty, low in calories (about 80 per egg), and filled with satisfying protein that helps curb cravings. In fact, it's a shame to eat them only at breakfast.

This egg salad recipe, a zesty twist on a classic, offers a healthy new way to work eggs into lunchtime. The low-fat Greek yogurt used in place of mayo dials down the fat and calories, while the curry powder provides a jolt of antioxidants.

Ingredients:

- 2 hard-cooked eggs, chopped

- 2 tablespoons plain Greek-style low-fat yogurt

- 2 tablespoons chopped red bell pepper

- 1/4 teaspoon curry powder

- 1/8 teaspoon salt

- 1/8 teaspoon pepper

- 2 slices rye bread, toasted

- 1/2 cup fresh spinach

- 1 orange

Preparation:

1. Combine eggs, yogurt, bell pepper, curry powder, salt, and pepper,

in a small bowl; stir well.

2. Place spinach on rye bread, top with egg salad, and serve the

orange on the side.

Nutritional Information:

Calories per serving:	410
Fat per serving:	14g
Saturated fat per serving:	4g
Monounsaturated fat per serving:	5g
Polyunsaturated fat per serving:	2g

Protein per serving: **22g**

Carbohydrate per serving: **51g**

Fiber per serving: **8g**

Cholesterol per serving: **425mg**

Sodium per serving: **870mg**

Resistant starch per serving: **1.8g**

Staying fit and healthy is a dynamic procedure since it is continually evolving. With exercise and all work-out activities we must focus on our diet, number of meals we are taking in a day and their proportions etc.

Those of you who are involved in consistent physical action do as much workout to improvise the present and future level of your health. We endeavor toward an ideal condition of prosperity. As our way of life enhances, our fitness additionally enhances and we encounter less ailment and infection. At the point when majority of people are questioned about their fitness they usually react with the four constituents of fitness said before (cardiorespiratory capacity, solid capacity, adaptability, and body synthesis).

Despite the fact that these segments are a basic part of being solid, they are not by any means the only contributing components. Physical wellbeing is standing out part of our general wellbeing.

Alternate segments of wellbeing (Greenberg, 2004, p. 7) that are generally as imperative as physical wellbeing incorporate the accompanying:

- Mental wellbeing the capacity to learn and become mentally. Backgrounds and in addition more formal structures (e.g., school) improve psychological well-being

- Emotional wellbeing the capacity to control feelings with the goal that you feel great communicating them and can express them properly.

- Social wellbeing the capacity to collaborate well with individuals and the earth and to have fulfilling individual connections.

- Spiritual wellbeing a confidence in some binding together compel. It shifts from individual to individual yet has the idea of confidence at its center.

Fitness is the quest for improved personal satisfaction, self-awareness, and potential through constructive way of life practices and states of mind. In the event that we assume liability for our own particular wellbeing and prosperity, we can enhance our wellbeing regularly. Certain variables impact our condition of wellbeing, including nourishment, physical movement, stress-adapting strategies, great connections, and profession achievement.

Every day we move in the direction of amplifying our level of wellbeing and to live long, full, and sound lives. The quest for fitness, self-awareness, and enhanced personal satisfaction depends on carrying on with a healthy lifestyle. To accomplish parity, we have to nurture our brain, body, and soul.

If these three regions are not working in proper coordination or disregarded, a person won't be at our ideal level of wellbeing. We are continually tested with adjusting each of these three zones all through life.

Experts or trainers of the field they have an obligation to manage and rouse others to enhance their level of wellbeing and health. You can elevate an all encompassing way to deal with your fitness (brain, body, and soul), not simply energize physical action. As great good examples, you ought to exhibit positive health practices that help with enhancing one's own wellbeing. In the event that your emphasis is entirely on the physical advantages of activity, you are doing a damage to our customers and you are not satisfying our expert commitment.

Some important guidelines for health:

• Endurance-On 4 to 7 days a week, perform constant movement for your heart, lungs, and circulatory framework. Time required for enhancements relies on upon exertion.

• Flexibility-On 4 to 7 days a week, perform tender achieving, twisting, and extending to keep muscles loose and joints flexible.

• Strength-On 2 to 4 days a week, perform resistance activity to fortify muscles and bones and enhance stamina.

• Perform 30 minutes or a greater amount of moderate-power physical movement on most days of the week for cardiovascular wellbeing. The 30 minutes need not be consistent.

• Performing 1 set of 8 to 12 redundancies of resistance preparing for the whole body is important to keep up and create strong quality and perseverance.

• Flexibility preparing ought to be performed day by day, including extends for all significant muscle bunches, keeping in mind the end goal to look after versatility.

Conclusion:

Concluding my text I would suggest that in this modern era there is a lot of knowledge available on internet as well as told through programs on TV. So we cannot say that we don't have proper guideline. We have all the tools available the only thing we lack is consistency and motivation. These both attributes comes when you are mentally and physically agreed to make your diet proper and keep your body in shape.

Different machines belts and other exercise equipment are easily available to public. You can join gym or you can set up a small gym of your own in your room or store room and you will experience the best body fitness. Try to do work-out with a friend or a family member this will keeps you motivated and you two can compete with each other on positive grounds, challenging yourselves to perform better than the other.

Nearly every one of you can be benefited from reducing the amount of unhealthy fat in your diet. If you are foodie and eat lots of fat, you should try these tips. If you implement two or even one of the following improvements you will be fascinated by its results:

- Instead of frying the meat. Try to bake, boil broil it. Peel off the skin and unnecessary fats on meat. Try to use chemical free meat. Make it a habit to eat fish at least once in a week.

- Try to reduce or cut down the additional fats. Instead of using butter or margarine as spread with bread in breakfast, us fruit jam or chutney. Try to use fresh vegetables or syrups for dressing instead of potato slices or cream dressing. Use low-fats for toppings.

- Try to maintain a kitchen garden so that you have fresh seasonal vegetables free of chemical to use in your meal. Eat salads as snack or even with meals.

- Avoid bakery items as much as possible. Cream dressings, cholate pastries and donuts are the source of excess fats you are carrying. Even during the travel try to satisfy your appetite with seasonal fruits and juices.

- Make it a habit to read nutrients proportion per serving when purchasing any readymade eatable.

- For drinks you should consume low-calorie drinks like water or unsweetened tea. Sweetened and fizzy drinks like instant energy drinks, organic juices, sports drinks, fruit drinks, soda, caffeinated drinks, frosted coffee or tea may include lots of calories and to your meal.

Be your own inspiration. This will not only makes you look fresh but you will also avoid many diseases. Nowadays people are dying in their early sixties and most deaths are reported to occur due to heart strokes. We can only avoid these by avoiding fats and other harmful foods in our diets. We need to avoid junk food and fizzy drinks. If we

eliminate these from our food we will surely be living happier, long

and anxiety free life.

I hope this book will inspire you and you will strive your level best to

avoid obesity and to stay healthy. Stay happy, stay fit.